YOUR THOUGHT AFFECTS YOUR EMOTION:

A perfect guide on how to deal with your emotions and feelings

Linda J.Barnes

Table of contents

Chapter 1

What are emotions?

Emotions have been concentrated on a few logical disciplines e.g., science, brain research, neuroscience, psychiatry, human studies, and social science as well as in business the executives, publicizing, and correspondences. Subsequently, unmistakable points of view on feeling have arisen, fitting to the intricacy and assortment of the actual feelings. It is significant, in any case, to take those alternate points of view not as cutthroat but rather as correlative, each possibly yielding understanding into what might be known as the unique "structures" of emotion. To say that feelings have structures (or a design) is to dismiss the view that they are simply nebulous "sentiments" or that they have no organization, rationale, or soundness. In actuality, emotions are organized in more than one way: by their basic nervous system science, by the decisions and assessments that go into them, by the way of behaving that communicates or shows them, and by the bigger social settings in which they happen. Hence, it could be said that an inclination is a "coordinated neuro-physiological-conduct evaluative-experiential-social peculiarity." Different feelings will show such designs to various degrees and in various ways, contingent upon the particular inclination, its sort, and the conditions.

In the rest of this article the designs of the various feelings will be viewed under three headings (however it ought to be borne as a main priority that the designs of any inclination are constantly coordinated into a natural entire): (1) actual designs, including the obvious way of behaving, nervous system science, and physiology; (2) experiential designs, or how an inclination is capable by the subject; and (3) social designs, including social causes and conditions, the social significance and capability of close to home articulations, the social impacts of a profound way of behaving, the political circumstances and results of profound way of behaving, and the moral contemplations that decide the nature and propriety of emotions.

Actual designs of emotions
During the principal half of the twentieth hundred years, individuals from the mental school of behaviorism endeavored to concentrate on mental peculiarities stringently concerning their freely discernible circumstances and results. As indicated by behaviorists, any truly logical record of feelings should be restricted to a depiction of the recognizable conditions that inspire feelings (the "upgrade") and the discernible actual changes and conduct that outcome from them (the "reaction"), including a particularly verbal way of behaving. Although behaviorism is not generally

viewed as a practical methodology, it ought to be noted exactly how much the component of the freely perceptible envelopes. The upgrade and reaction circumstances incorporate not just the actual environmental elements of individuals encountering the inclination and any development, signal, or sound they make yet, in addition, their neurological,neurochemical,physiological states including, for instance, chemical levels and varieties in the movement of the autonomic sensory system, which controls and manages interior organs.

The neurobiology of emotion
Before the coming of behaviorism, when the study of nervous system science was still in its early stages, the American thinker and analyst William James (1842-1910) brought a portion of the variables together in his hypothesis of feeling, which he set out in his central review The Principles of Psychology

(1890). In about a couple dozen pages, James referred to a wide assortment of physiological changes engaged with certain feelings: autonomic sensory system action (hustling heart, expansion of the veins, tightening of the bladder and entrails, compulsory changes in breathing, and "something in the pharynx that propels either a swallow, a getting free from the throat, or a slight hack"), trademark "profound" mental processes, "anxious expectations," and plain actual articulations and activities shudder, sobbing, running, and striking. For James, such feelings are actual impressions that go with specific physiological changes that themselves are achieved by some "disturbing" discernment. Likewise, in a well-known suggestion, he encouraged the people who wished to work on their profound state to "smooth the forehead, light up the eye, contract the dorsal as opposed to the ventral part of the casing, and talk in a significant key, and pass the warm commendation.

Research has since recognized the substantial changes considered by James. Autonomic sensory system action, which is some of the time taken to be the center of James' hypothesis, is unmistakable from deliberate muscle movement. Contemporary nervous system science has come to zero in substantially more on cerebrum action accordingly and to regard any remaining substantial changes as strictly optional. Neuroscientific research has shown not just that feelings have their beginnings in brain activity in the mind but that various feelings show different examples of brain action. The center of profound cerebrum action is by all accounts the limbic forebrain: the thalamus, the nerve center, the reticular development, and the amygdala, which are all subcortical (beneath the cerebral cortex). The nerve center has significant connections to joy and wretchedness,while the reticular arrangement might have a significant connection to discouragement.The American neuroscientist Joseph E. LeDoux has shown that the hear-able feeling of dread includes the transmission of sound signs through the heart-able pathway to the thalamus (which transfers data) and afterward to the dorsal amygdala (which assesses data). Such examination recommends that feeling that is actuated via the thalamo-amygdala pathway results from evaluative handling that is quick, negligible, and programmed. In any case, feeling may likewise be enacted through a hand-off of data from the thalamus to the neocortex (the external piece of the cerebral cortex), and this circuit is the brain's reason for mental examination and assessment of occasions. Accordingly, there are two brain connections associated with the actuation of emotion: cortical and subcortical. The initiation of feeling through the thalamo-amygdala pathway makes sense of how babies and extremely small kids answer genuinely to agony and why grown-ups' areas of strength express and cause profound decisions before they have any cognizant acknowledgment of doing such. Individuals frequently experience feelings before they structure explanations behind having the emotions they do.

The two sides of the equator of the cerebrum are connected diversely to profound cycles. The right side of the equator might be more capable than the left at separating between profound articulations. Additionally, it has been contended that the right side of the equator might be more associated with handling pessimistic feelings, and the left half of the globe is more associated with handling good feelings. Individuals who are restless, furious, or discouraged show expanded action in the amygdala and the right prefrontal cortex. Individuals feeling good show expanded action in the left prefrontal cortex, while the amygdala and the right prefrontal cortex stay calm. The vast majority experience the two kinds of states of mind and feelings, however, people likewise appear to have a pretty much fixed natural inclination to be content or to be restless. Indeed, even after favorable luck or horrible luck, individuals, at last, will quite often get back to their normal day-to-day mindsets. (There is some proof, notwithstanding, that activities like contemplation can move a common state of mind toward the positive.) Over the years there have been different speculations about precisely where the brain bases of a feeling lie. Yet, the most conceivable hypotheses demand that mind capabilities overall include complex communications between various parts; subsequently, the journey to the "middle" of feeling might be off track.

The accentuation of the job of the cerebrum in feeling raises the proposition of the characteristic of profound responses, which was safeguarded by Charles Darwin (1809-82) as well as by James. A few contemporary hypotheses contend that feelings, or if nothing else the "essential" feelings, are established in a person's natural cosmetics and that qualities are huge determinants of the limit and trademark power level of every fundamental inclination. Different hypotheses guarantee that hereditary variables are immaterial and that feelings are intellectually developed or obtained for a fact, particularly from socialization and learning (see underneath Social designs of emotions). In any case, close-to-home life is a component of the collaboration of hereditary propensities and the evaluative convictions procured through experience. This incorporates even the essential feelings, which might well have an innate neurological center yet manifest themselves just inside the social requirements given by social experience.

In an early human turn of events, most feelings and their demeanors get from programmed, subcortical handling, with a negligible cortical contribution. As mental limits increase with development and learning, the neocortex and the cortico-amygdala pathway become progressively more included. When kids gain language and the limit with regards to long haul memory, they might handle occasions in one or the other or the two pathways, with the subcortical pathway spending significant time in occasions requiring quick reaction and the cortico-amygdala pathway giving evaluative data important to mental judgment and more complicated survival methods.

The actual articulation of emotion

There has been a lot of exploration on close-to-home articulation, especially on those articulations that are generally quick, generally obvious, and normally generally unconstrained or programmed and consequently frequently obscure to the subject who shows them. Darwin noticed the striking comparability between the close-to-home articulations of numerous well-evolved creatures and people; he consequently hypothesized both a developmental clarification of the likeness and an anthropological proposition that looks of feeling, like those of outrage, shock, and dread, are widespread in people. During the 1960s the American analyst Paul Ekman set off to discredit Darwin's anthropological proposition however found, to his underlying shock, that it was affirmed by mounting multifaceted proof. From that point forward, investigations of the trademark looks of different feelings and their acknowledgment have been a prevailing subject of mental examination. Not all feelings have trademark looks, obviously, thus studies will generally focus upon a little arrangement of fundamental feelings e.g., outrage, disdain, dread, euphoria, bitterness, and shock. Every one of these feelings, as indicated by numerous scholars, comprises an "influence program" , a complicated arrangement of looks, vocalizations, and autonomic and skeletal reactions. It is as yet a question of discussion whether feelings that are probably fundamental can be caught as far as influence programs; in this manner, it is likewise disputable whether the acknowledgment and creation of normal looks are for sure general and "designed."

One of the captivating highlights of unconstrained looks is how troublesome it is for a great many people to "counterfeit" a genuine articulation. This is maybe most clear on account of grinning (as a statement of joy or being satisfied). Clinicians have long perceived the Duchenne grin (named for the French nervous system specialist Guillaume-Benjamin-AmandDuchenne [1806-75]), an earnest and unconstrained grin that is described by the extending of the mouth as well as by the rise of the cheeks and the particular constriction of the muscles around the eye. In a bogus or non-Duchenne grin, these different components are missing and, hence, it is not difficult to perceive a misleading grin regardless of whether one has no clue about what it is that parts with it.

The conduct articulation of feeling likewise incorporates cognizant and oblivious motions, stances and quirks, and a clear way of behaving that can be either unconstrained or purposeful. One could wonder whether or not to consider a purposeful way of behaving an "articulation" on account of the mediating cognizant action it includes. One could talk rather than such a way of behaving as being "out of" the inclination (as in, "he carried on outrage"). However, the contrast between the two cases is much of the time extremely slight. Carrying on of outrage might be prompt, as on account of an unconstrained affront, or it could be extended or postponed. It might very well be communicated in a progression of correctional activities that happen for months or years or in wrathful demonstrations that follow the inciting event and the outrage by a similarly extended timeframe. However, even the quick articulation of feeling in clear activity might be (and typically is) extended in time and not only transitory. Running from risk in dread might happen however long it needs to (as long as the danger is obvious). The outflow of significant love, many individuals would agree, happens for a lifetime, however it might likewise comprise of quite a few both unconstrained and conscious demonstrations and signals.

Verbal articulations are quite compelling. They can be unconstrained and prompt, similar to the hoots and cheers of avid supporters, yet they can be more smooth, articulate, and purposeful. A memorial service discourse might be genuine and expressive of the feeling of melancholy; a conciliatory sentiment can likewise be sincere and expressive of the feelings of disgrace and regret. Furthermore, the recitation of an affection sonnet can act as a sweeping "I love you."

Experiential designs of emotion
James presented his hypothesis of feelings with a significant capability: "I ought to express most importantly that the main feelings I propose explicitly to consider here are those that have an unmistakable substantial articulation." Although there are

feelings that have no such articulation, James demanded that all feelings have a psychological or cognizant aspect.

The starting reason for feeling, as per James, is an insight. James didn't take discernment to be a constituent of feeling, however, he perceived its significance. To place the matter such that he didn't, James perceived that an inclination should be "tied in with" something. It isn't simply an inclination in light of a physiological aggravation. James suggested deliberateness, the component of a few mental cycles in the goodness of which they are basically about or coordinated toward an item. Numerous scholars following James have modified his investigation by including insight and its purposefulness, as a fundamental piece of feeling. For sure, a few scholars have guaranteed that an inclination is only an extraordinary sort of insight. The idea of close-to-home insight, likewise, has been significantly improved to incorporate not just actual impressions of what is happening in one's body yet additionally perceptual encounters of what is happening in the world. In the investigation of feeling, that viewpoint is a close-to-home viewpoint, "hued" by the different feelings as well as by the novel point of view of the subject. In any case, the normal allegory of variety doesn't do equity to close-to-home insight. The feeling isn't something unmistakable and some way or another overlays an encounter; the experience is essential for the design of the actual feeling.

The experiential designs of feeling incorporate, most importantly, deliberateness and what's going on with the inclination — an individual, a demonstration, an occasion, or a situation. Yet, deliberateness is organized thus by the subject's convictions and evaluative decisions about the individual, act, occasion, or situation being referred to. The significance of faith in feeling has provoked numerous scholars to plan "mental" speculations of feeling, while an accentuation on assessment has driven others to figure out "evaluation" hypotheses. Such hypotheses are much of the time the same, changing mostly in their accentuation of the essential significance of conviction rather than evaluative judgment. They don't challenge the significance of what is, for the most part, alluded to as "feeling" in feeling, however, they do make the idea of those sentiments substantially more mind-boggling and fascinating than in the Jamesian view. Feelings include information, convictions, sentiments, and wants about the world. Hence, the feeling should incorporate material sentiments as well as the intellectually rich encounters of knowing, drawing in, and being mindful.

The experiential component of an inclination incorporates actual sensations as well as the experience of an item and its current circumstance through the remarkable viewpoint given by that inclination. The experience of being angry at Smith, for instance, comprises generally the experience of Smith according to a specific point of view e.g., as being hostile, disdainful, or meriting discipline. The experience of being enamored with Jones comprises generally in the experience of Jones according to another viewpoint e.g., as being adorable, extraordinary, or remarkably meriting care. The encounters of outrage and cherish likewise incorporate different contemplations and recollections and goals to act in some ways.

The profound experience likewise incorporates joy and torment, as Aristotle demanded, however seldom as segregated sentiments. On a more regular basis, various parts of an inclination are pleasurable or excruciating, as considerations or recollections might be pleasurable or difficult. The inclination as such might be pleasurable or excruciating (e.g., pride or regret), thus may one's affirmation of the way that one has a specific inclination (charmed to be enamored once more, annoyed with oneself for flying off the handle or desirous). Yet, once more, profound issues are not generally so clear. It is normal to have "blended feelings," when the counter currents of delight and agony make it hard to choose a solitary perspective.

Social designs of emotion
Even though Darwin felt that close to home articulations are because of "the constitution of the sensory system" and assume a part in transformation and endurance, he accepted that others fill an alternate need: the

correspondence of feeling to other people. For sure, the omnipresence and consistency of looks of feeling would be difficult to understand if it were not for the way that they impart a singular's feelings to different individuals from his gathering or species. By grinning one shows neighborliness and maybe an absence of expectation to hurt; by scowling one conveys the inverse. The profound looks that are so obvious in the face and body act as the principal method for correspondence between a mother and her baby. As Darwin noted, "We promptly see compassion in others by their appearance; our sufferings are consequently alleviated. We chuckle together and our shared pleasantness increases and reinforces our pleasure." The social part of the feeling, appropriately, is most clear in broad daylight showcases feelings, which straightforwardly influence the way of behaving of others. Be that as it may, this angle incorporates significantly more than correspondence. It additionally incorporates the social constitution, or social development, of feelings with and through others. The social designs of feeling comprise the manners by which the bigger social setting decides an inclination's causes, content, methods of articulation, and importance. Indeed, even the fundamental feelings, which are for the most part expected to have a neurological center, are molded generally by friendly elements.

Social setting decides the reasons for feelings from a conspicuous perspective: various conditions incite various feelings in various societies. A Vodou (Voodoo) revile, for instance, produces fear in one society but just bemusement in another. A spouse who sees his significant other in the organization of another man becomes desirous in one society but might be detached in another. All feelings include insight, and all are impacted by virtues and evaluative ideas, many (while perhaps not) of which are all educated. The ideas of good and bad, fitting and unseemly, and their legitimate application are learned in the particular conditions of each gathering or society.

Nervous system

Human nervous system: Emotion and conduct

To complete the right way of behaving in other words, right comparable to the endurance of the individual.

Feelings are dependent upon social forming in their methods of articulation as in many articulations, maybe even those that are pretty much designed, are dependent upon neighborhood "show rules," which administer which feelings and which articulations are suitable in which conditions. An outflow of outrage is improper in most open conditions in Japan, however, it is very normal at a metropolitan crossing point in the United States. The social significance of an inclination is additionally (and) not set in stone. In Tahiti outrage is viewed as very hazardous and is even disparaged; in the Mediterranean it is in many cases an indication of virility, proposing honesty. It is not necessarily the case that the social effects on feeling are restricted to their social understandings. The actual feelings are, in some measure to a limited extent, of such understandings. The socially comprised piece of an inclination might be more modest in essential feelings than in intellectually rich feelings like moral resentment and heartfelt love, however, culture as well as science, social contrasts as well as individual contrasts, figure out what feelings there are and whether, where, and when having them is proper.

The way that emotions include conduct, considerations, and culture brings up the issue of whether or how much feelings are objective. For logicians like Plato (c. 428-c. 348 BCE) and David Hume (1711-76), who imagined feeling and sanity as clashing contrary energies, such an inquiry was improper all along. However, conduct and contemplations can be reasonable or nonsensical, and culture forces its principles of soundness. To that degree, in any event, clear profound articulations and contemplations can be decided by such principles. Out of resentment, individuals frequently act and think unreasonably. Yet, what is on rare occasions accentuated is that outrage can bring about conduct and considerations that are very normal, as in they are decisively fruitful in articulating or directing the feeling into useful activity. The contemplations that one has out of frustration may likewise be precise and smart — e.g., recollecting past insults and an example of a hostile way of behaving. Also, culture forces its own rules for concluding which articulations and considerations are reasonable, as well as which feelings having in which circumstances are normal. To be desirous in specific societies and specific conditions might be completely fitting and along these lines reasonable. Be that as it may, in different societies or different conditions desire is improper and in this manner silly.

An inclination can likewise be objective or nonsensical in two additional particulars detected: (1) it tends to be pretty much exactly in the discernment or comprehension of the circumstance it includes; and (2) it very well may be pretty much justified in its assessment of the circumstance. An illustration of (1) is: Smith resents Jones for offering something hostile when Jones said nothing of the sort and there is not a glaringly obvious explanation to feel that he did. An illustration of (2) is: Smith resents Jones for offering something hostile, however as a matter of fact what Jones said was not hostile since it was not purposeful or because it was a precise and useful analysis of Smith, for which Smith ought not to be irritated or furious. In the primary model, the outrage is nonsensical because it depends on deception about the circumstance; in the subsequent, it is unreasonable because it includes an uncalled for or out-of-line assessment.

In one more sense, feelings can be objective to the extent that they are useful. It has become something of a saying in contemporary brain science that feelings have developed alongside people and are in this manner the result of normal choice. It doesn't follow, notwithstanding, that a specific inclination was separately chosen for, or that feelings serve, the capabilities that might have made them important previously. Outrage might have been a valuable improvement of hostility in ancient times, yet it tends to be malicious or for the most part broken in a cutting-edge metropolitan climate. Additionally, feelings (or specific feelings) likely could be side-effects of other developed qualities. In any case, when in doubt, feelings truly do assume a significant part in individuals' private and public activities. For sure, Hume demanded that an explanation without help from anyone else gives no inspiration to a moral way of behaving; just feelings can do that. Current neuroscience has reached a lot of a similar end.

At long last, emotions s can be sane as in they can be utilized to accomplish specific essential human objectives and goals. Lashing out might be a significant stage in propelling oneself to confront obstructions and defeat them. Experiencing passionate feelings might be a significant stage in fostering the ability to frame and keep up with personal connections. All the same, lashing out at one's supervisor might be entirely justified yet unreasonable to the extent that it disappoints one's vocation objectives. A Buddhist priest might be completely legitimate in being desirous of an individual priest, yet his envy is in any case silly to the extent that it is contrary to his origination of himself as a Buddhist. In this sense, feelings give both the substance of a decent life and its finishes. Along these lines, the French existentialist rationalist Jean-Paul Sartre (1905-80) contended that feelings are systems. Individuals use them to control others and, more significantly, to move into perspectives and acting that suit their objectives and their mental self-view.

Since emotions are the item of culture as well as one's way of behaving and perspectives after some time, one is partially answerable for them. Emotions can be deliberately evolved or deterred via preparing oneself to respond pretty much sincerely — or with a greater amount of one sort of feeling and less of another — in specific conditions. For Aristotle, this sort of preparation is important for the most common way of developing a decent upright person in oneself. Having the right feelings in the perfect sums and the right conditions, as he contended, is the pith of temperance and the way to human prospering.

Chapter 2

How are emotions formed?

The Theory of Constructed Emotion offers an extremist new interpretation of what emotions are, where they come from, and how they shape our lives.

Introduced by brain research teacher and neuroscientist Dr. Lisa Feldman Barrett in her smash hit book How Emotions Are Made (subsidiary connection), it likewise goes against a significant number of our most immovably held thoughts regarding how human emotions work.

For instance, that's what it contends:

Emotions are not permanently set up in an old, "reptilian" part of the cerebrum

Emotions can't be identified through looks or some other physiological estimation

There are no "all inclusive" emotions across individuals, countries, or societies

There are no particular pieces of the mind devoted to explicit emotions (like the amygdala for dread)

Emotions are not "responses" to outside occasions

Throughout recent years, Dr. Barrett and her group at the Interdisciplinary Affective Science Laboratory at Northeastern University have jabbed and pushed the faces, bodies, and minds of thousands of subjects, attempting to open the insider facts about the profound cerebrum.

In this article, I'll sum up the fundamental thoughts from the book to assist them with spreading as all over as could be expected. Expect all that beneath is straightforwardly taken or reworded from the book, although I've attempted to make sense of it as would be natural for me. Any mix-ups or misinterpretations are mine.

Emotions are ideas

The Theory of Constructed Emotion takes its name from its focal reason: that emotions are ideas that are developed by the mind.

Think about your cerebrum briefly. It's staying there in your skull, getting a wide range of information from your eyes, ears, nose, skin, and mouth. This information is educational, yet in addition vague. It must be deciphered.

For instance, it could think:

What is that rectangular wellspring of light with changing examples of variety? A window!

What is this irregular example of little, cool spots clearing across my body? Downpour!

What is that musical example of gaseous tension changes? A melody

Along these lines, the mind is continually attempting to figure out the information it is getting. One of the least demanding ways for it to do that is to involve previous experience as an aide. On the off chance that it can coordinate the ongoing involvement in memory, it can save a ton of significant investment.

Be that as it may, it would take excessively lengthy for it to think about a great many old recollections, each in turn.

All things being equal, the mind utilizes ideas. An idea resembles a compacted form of hundreds or thousands of previous encounters. Rather than recollecting each experience you've at any point had with a "seat," for instance, your cerebrum stores an idea of a seat. The following time you experience a seat, your mind just needs to coordinate it with this idea for it to comprehend how the situation is playing out.

Ideas are like names or classifications that your mind has made to get a handle on your general surroundings. When you see a novel, a new thing, your mind doesn't inquire "What is this?"; it inquires "How is this?". As such, your mind is continually attempting to put all that you see into a current classification. This is a lot simpler than attempting to sort out what it is without any preparation.

The possibility that we use ideas to get a handle on our experience isn't new. Be that as it may, Emotions like "dread," "trouble," and "dissatisfaction" are ideas very much like some others. Similarly, as your cerebrum deciphers an example of light as a "window," it could decipher an example of substantial sensations as "dread" or "frustration." These emotions don't feel like ideas since we experience them with a burning intensity. In any case, they are.

To act as an illustration of how this functions, Dr. Barrett recounts the tale of watching the report about a new school shooting. It felt at the time like she was responding straightforwardly to the news. She felt awful pain and misery, and tears appeared to come suddenly to her eyes.

However, it would be more exact to depict what happened this way:

"I learned quite a while in the past that "misery" is something that might happen when certain substantial sentiments harmonize with horrendous misfortune. Utilizing pieces and bits of previous experience, for example, my insight into shootings and my past trouble with them, my mind quickly anticipated how my body ought to adapt to such misfortune. Its forecasts caused my pounding heart, my flushed face, and the bunches in my stomach. They guided me to cry, an activity that would quiet my sensory system. What's more, they made the subsequent sensations significant as an occurrence of misery."

All in all, her experience of bitterness was a "reenactment" or expectation of the suitable way for her body to respond to the news. The misery was not an unadulterated response to something occurring outwardly. It rose out of a perplexing transaction of frameworks making an inevitable expectation about what was required for her body to adapt.

Emotions are predictions
Since the mind isn't inactively noticing approaching information from the rest of the world. That would settle on its exceptionally sluggish choices, possibly undermining our endurance.

To act all the more rapidly, the cerebrum begins responding even before it has gotten every one of the information - it makes a "reproduction" or forecast of its thought process that could occur straight away. Fundamentally, the cerebrum is continually making its most realistic estimation of what its thought process is going to happen and afterward planning to follow up on that conjecture.

Assuming your cerebrum surmises that you are playing soccer, for instance, it could begin anticipating a wide range of likely situations in light of previous experience: potential chances to run for the objective, quick balls flying toward your head, or approaching assailants from any course. The cerebrum could begin setting up the body for these situations somewhat early, by diverting the bloodstream to specific muscles or turning out to be more careful about flying soccer balls.

The same thing occurs with absolutely mental exercises. As you read this text at the present moment, your cerebrum is foreseeing which word or thought is probably going to come straight away, in view that could only be described as an epic of understanding experience. These forecasts save energy and assist you with perusing quicker than would some way or another be conceivable. As the biggest and most energy-hungry organ in the body, the mind enormously focuses on this proficiency.

What's more, the same interaction occurs with our emotions. En route to the air terminal to get a companion you haven't seen for a long time, your mind is occupied with anticipating the sensations of delight and bliss you will before long be feeling. And that implies you are now feeling cheerful before the occasion has happened, and feel significantly more joyful when you see her.

The expectation is such a basic movement of the human mind that a few researchers think of it as the cerebrum's default method of activity. Your mind can't resist the urge to continually fabricate prescient models of every experience you have or any experience it figures you could have.

This prompts a significant end: that the reenactments we make in our minds are more genuine to us than the actual world. What we see, hear, contact, taste, and smell are recreations of the world, not responses to it. We could believe that our view of the world is driven by occasions on the planet, however, a large portion of what we see depends on our inner expectations. The information rolling in from our faculties simply impacts our discernments, similar to a little stone skirting across a moving sea wave.

This alarming end is supported by research on how people see. The piece of the mind liable for sight, the visual cortex, gets just 10% of its associations from the retina. The other 90% are associations from different pieces of the mind, making expectations about how the situation is playing out.

How does the mind respond when its expectations are off-base? It can change its forecast to match everything the faculties are saying to it. However, doing the inverse: staying with the first forecast, and channeling the approaching information so it matches the prediction is similarly possible.

One might say, your mind is wired for hallucination: you experience your very own intricate universe creation, which is kept within proper limits by pieces of tactile information. When your forecasts are sufficiently right, they channel your discernment and figure out what you're ready to find in any case. This can turn into a shut circle where the mind just sees what it accepts, and afterward accepts what it sees.

According to the mind's perspective, the body is simply one more piece of the outside world that it should make sense of. Furthermore, it utilizes the same system we just analyzed to decipher sensations coming from inside the body - the changing rhythms of your pulse, the sensation of breathing, the thundering of your stomach, and the constriction and widening of your veins.

It's essential to comprehend that these actual sensations from inside the body have no goal meaning. They feel so extraordinary because they're coming from inside you. Be that as it may, a hurt in your stomach, for instance, could straightforwardly be "made sense of" as:

Hunger (assuming that you're finding a spot during supper)
Looming ailment (assuming it's influenza season)
Shock (if you are going through a separation)
A conviction that a litigant is conniving (if you're an appointed authority in a court and haven't eaten)
The method involved in deciphering these real sensations is called interoception. It is overseen by an "interoceptive organization"

in the mind that learns from your inner organs and tissues, the chemicals in your blood, and your resistant framework, among numerous others, and marks this data with an idea, for example, "yearning" or "disaster." These emotions might feel like they are coming straightforwardly from your body. In any case, they are being built by the interoceptive organization in your mind, dependent generally upon your expectations.

What is the reason for interoception?
All that your body does, inside or out, requires energy. To deal with its "body financial plan" across many body parts and billions of cells, the mind needs to continually anticipate the body's energy needs. Similarly, as a money division needs a financial plan to conjecture where cash will be required, the mind makes forecasts and issues rectifications about when and where it figures energy will be required.

Large numbers of these "monetary changes" we experience as profound encounters. Your muscles running nearly out of energy could feel like "weariness." Too little rest may be deciphered as "overpower." An absence of good friendly cooperation may be capable of "dejection." But these emotions are not objective realities. They are ideas worked by the brain out of bits of tactile information, social information, and a past filled with social connections. Interoception was developed to adjust our body spending plans. Encountering emotions is a lucky (and here and there lamentable) secondary effect.

The fact that there is something off-base makes this implies a "terrible inclination" proof. It simply implies you are burdening your body spending plan. Emotions are genuine, yet everything that they appear to be saying to you isn't genuine. Knowing that "pessimistic" emotions are just our cerebrum's approach to letting us know that stores are running short, we can settle on purposeful choices to top off those stores, rather than going after less solid survival techniques.

Experiential visual deficiency
Indeed, even with all the logical proof on the planet, it tends to be truly challenging to accept that emotions are inside-produced ideas driven by mental recreations. They feel so extraordinary and overpowering at the time, similar to a wave clearing us away despite our desire to the contrary.

The explanation that emotions feel like responses to things occurring in the rest of the world has to do with how ideas are utilized by the mind. Ideas are not simply names for the things we latently notice. They are important as far as we're concerned to see things in any case. An idea fills in as a focal point (or some of the time, a channel) for what we can find in any case.

Imagine you are sitting in a Parisian bistro as an extended get-away, tasting fine wine and eating cheddar. You might hear a French couple at the following table over-drenched in a discussion. The discussion contains all the data you would have to comprehend what they're talking about. However, if your brain is feeling the loss of a bunch of ideas known as "the French language," it will sound useless to you.

This is known as "experiential visual deficiency" - the powerlessness to see what you don't as of now have an idea for. Recall that we are not encountering the world straightforwardly; we are encountering our psychological recreation of it. What's more, without an idea for something, we can't integrate it into our reproduction

Our ideas permit us to see things in a world that generally gives just deficient, uncertain data. They assist us with perceiving things rapidly and (normally) precisely while saving investment. Yet, the most common way of utilizing ideas to see things occurs so undetectably and naturally, that our faculties can feel like reflexes as opposed to developments. We feel no feeling of organization for the reenactments we are running.

This makes sense of why an inclination like "joy" can feel like it's a response to outside occasions, instead of being created from inside the mind. Indeed, even before your cerebrum has wrapped up classifying what is happening as "bliss," it is additionally recreating satisfaction ahead of time. Outer discernment meets interior development before you understand what's going on, so it appears as though joy is occurring to you when your cerebrum is effectively building the experience.

This can likewise turn into an inevitable forecast: the more you anticipate that satisfaction should show up, the more arrangements you make for its appearance, and the more probable you are to encounter it. Indeed, even on a neurological level, you make your existence.

The significance of close-to-home granularity One of the most difficult ramifications of the Theory of Constructed Emotions is that, on the off chance that somebody doesn't have an idea to depict an inclination, they will not have the option to see it. They'll in any case feel the substantial sensations

Envision an outrageous model: somebody who just can't recognize "great" and "terrible" sentiments. They show low profound granularity. Since they have just lose data about what's going on inside their bodies, it will be hard for such an individual to deal with a considerable lot of life's difficulties. They will be experientially ignorant concerning even their sentiments.

This represents the basic significance of high profound granularity. Getting a handle on substantial sensations requires energy, and attempting to sort a gigantic measure of tangible information into an expansive inclination like "satisfaction" takes a ton of energy. Presently suppose you had a more exact idea for the sensation of connection to a dear companion, for example, the Korean word Jeong (정). Your mind would require less work to develop this more tight idea. Accuracy prompts productivity; this is the natural result of higher close-to-home granularity.

At the point when you experience a feeling without knowing the exact reason, you are bound to regard that feeling as data about the world, instead of your experience of the world. This is known as emotional authenticity. Emotional authenticity makes us experience assumed "realities" about the world that are made by our sentiments. It can leave us caught in a close-to-home universe through our effort, without understanding that we are the ones who detained ourselves.

Fortunately, close-to-home granularity can be moved along. If you can figure out how to recognize more exact implications for "Feeling perfect" (cheerful, content, excited, loose, happy, confident, motivated, prideful, loving, appreciative, delighted . . .) or "Feeling awful" (irate, irritated, frightened, angry, surly, contrite, bleak, embarrassed, uncomfortable, fear-ridden, angry, apprehensive, desirous, sad, despairing . . .), your cerebrum will have a lot more choices for foreseeing, classifying, and seeing emotions.

High close-to-home granularity provides us with a lot more noteworthy scope of devices, permitting more adaptable reactions to our difficulties. It permits us to fit our activities to the hidden reasons for our emotions, instead of their nearby appearance.

Developing social reality

Although emotions are produced from the inside, they don't stop there. We use emotions to develop our social reality.

At the point when you cooperate with individuals you know and like - your life partner, companions, darlings, kids, colleagues, or close associates - you synchronize your pulses, breathing, and other actual signs, prompting quantifiable advantages. Something as straightforward as clasping hands with a friend or family member or keeping their image in front of you can further develop body planning and decrease torment. All in all, we additionally utilize others to control our body spending plans.

Be that as it may, this goes a long way past dealing with our body's financial plans. Ideas like "dread," "expectation," and "disdain" are ideas your mind uses to control others' bodies also. When we develop a feeling idea and name it with a word, we can impart it to other people, permitting them to see what we see and in this way reworking how their minds work. When you and I share an idea, I can only express a word to begin sending off expectations in your cerebrum, a sort of semantic clairvoyance.

Rather than a restricted arrangement of emotions worked in from birth, nature gave us the unrefined components to bootstrap a calculated framework, including feeling ideas. With input from the grown-ups who expressed feeling words to us purposefully and consciously, we acquired the capacity to see actual articles, yet thoughts that dwell just in the personalities of individuals: objectives, aims, inclinations, and their own emotions.

Over the long haul, this intergenerational move of feeling information - as stories, customs, fantasies, tales, or truly anything that we can impart - permits every age to shape the cerebrum wiring of the following. This group of information is the quintessence of our progress similarly as much as the books in our libraries.

Present-day culture and body spending plans When you comprehend body financial plans and what they mean for our emotions, it becomes obvious the amount of current culture appears to be designed to disturb them.

A large part of the food we eat is loaded with refined sugar that twists our body's financial plans. School and occupations make them wake early and nod off late, leaving the north of 40% of Americans somewhere in the range of 13 and 64 consistently sleepless, which prompts persistent mis budgeting. Publicists play on our uncertainties, recommending we'll be passed judgment on gravely by our companions if we don't look or purchase a specific way (and social dismissal is harmful to our body spending plans). Virtual entertainment offers many more open doors for social examination, while steady cell phone utilization implies we never genuinely unwind.

Recall that the whole experience of emotions depends on our cerebrum's expectations about what it thinks our body needs. Assuming that those expectations become constantly in conflict with our body's real necessities, it very well may be difficult to bring them back into balance. Your body spending plans don't answer effectively to advance notice signals from your body for what it's worth. When our expectations have been misguided for a considerable length of time, you will feel persistently hopeless without knowing why.

What do we do when we feel hopeless? We self-cure. About a third of all prescriptions consumed in the United States are taken to deal with some type of pain. We use liquor, medications, TV, and sugar to accomplish a similarity to spending plan balance, yet at a horrible expense of compulsion and stoutness. It has become clear in late many years that the safe framework affects undeniably a larger number of sicknesses and destructive circumstances than we envisioned, including diabetes, stoutness, coronary illness, gloom, a sleeping disorder, malignant growth, decreased memory, and other mental capabilities connected with untimely maturing and dementia. Furthermore, the insusceptible framework endures when our body's financial plans leave balance.

Looking all the more carefully at sadness gives a window into how persistently imbalanced body financial plans can have intensifying adverse consequences.

Wretchedness can be considered a persevering input circle of pessimistic considerations and sentiments. Each feeling drives the following idea, as well as the other way around. The mind harps on regrettable previous encounters, and subsequently continue to make withdrawals on a generally burdened spending plan. Caution signals from the body are turned down or overlooked. As a result, the body and brain are gotten into a pattern of uncorrected expectations, caught in an unfriendly past when metabolic requirements were high.

Since the body's financial plan is constantly in the red, the body attempts to cut spending. The simplest method for doing that is to quit moving around and quit focusing on the world. On the off chance that a discouraged individual begins keeping away from individuals, others can't assist with adjusting their body financial plan by the same token. This is the tenacious weakness of gloom.

This cycle additionally applies, obviously, to individuals who experience childhood misfortune, coming up short on fundamental necessities like security, food, and rest. These circumstances change the interoceptive organization, decreasing the mind's capacity to control its financial plan for life precisely.

This converts into a higher lifetime hazard of coronary illness, joint inflammation, diabetes, malignant growth, and different sicknesses.

Another interpretation of the moral obligation Considering the likelihood that we develop our emotions in light of ideas, the following inquiry is, would we say we are answerable for our ideas?

Not every one of them, positively. You can't pick the ideas you advanced as a kid. In any case, as a grown-up, you have options about what encounters you open yourself to, which shapes the ideas that at last drive your activities. Obligation, in this view, is tied in with pursuing purposeful decisions to change your ideas.

The Theory of Constructed Emotion contends that each part of our emotions is pliant and adaptable. You are not helpless before legendary inclination circuits are covered somewhere inside some antiquated piece of your mind. You have more command over your emotions than you naturally suspect.

You can't simply snap your fingers and immediately change what you're feeling, however the following are six functional advances you can take to work on your profound granularity over the long haul, in light of the latest discoveries from logical exploration.

1. Take a stab at new points of view
As per the Theory of Constructed Emotion, the ideas we hold straightforwardly influence our body's financial plans, and in this manner our experience of emotions. There is no such thing as ideas in a theoretical, rarified domain separate from science. Learning or evolving ideas (otherwise called mental models)

straightforwardly influences how our body works moment to minute.

By taking a stab at new points of view on how we take a stab at new garments, we can "test" different body-planning systems. In the same way, we could assign more monetary assets to some financial plan classification, we can do likewise with our body financial plans.

This can remember anything from a movement for far-off nations to investing energy with various types of individuals, to understanding writing, to attempting new encounters. These encounters open us to various approaches to addressing human necessities that we might need to get for ourselves.

2. Recategorize what you're feeling

Whenever you're feeling awful, perceive what is occurring: you are encountering horrendous influence in light of interoceptive sensations. With training, you can figure out how to dismantle the feeling into its constituent parts, rather than allowing it to turn into a focal point through which you view the world.

For instance, the expansive, equivocal sensation of "uneasiness" can be separated and recategorized into "strain across the upper back," "quickly thumping heart," and "grasped jaw." This deconstruction denies the vibes of a portion of their profound power.

Take a stab at naming what you are feeling all the more unequivocally, mulling over various pieces of the body, or searching for additional quick, actual causes like yearning, drying out, or absence of rest.

3. Discuss what you're feeling

One of the best approaches to scrutinizing the brain's in many cases excessively sensational understandings is

In examinations, men who communicated a ton of feelings that they didn't mark were found to have the most significant levels of cytokines, proteins that over the drawn-out cause irritation. Female bosom disease survivors who unequivocally name and express their emotions have better well-being and fewer clinical visits after a medical procedure.

This isn't cushioned self-improvement counsel: discussing your sentiments quantifiably works on your well-being and satisfaction.

4. Move your body

Now and again the prescient circles among body and brain areas of strength are to such an extent that it is hard to hinder them deliberately. Fortunately, we have a secondary passage: the body. Whether through strolling, yoga, extending, weight training, or different types of activity, we can re-synchronize the signs streaming between our body and brain, putting our body spending plans once again into balance.

All creatures use development to manage their body's financial plans. If a canine has an excess of glucose in its framework, it can go here and there aimlessly to consume it. People are special in that we can utilize mental ideas to move our financial plans. Yet, when that fizzles, a fast run or oxygen-consuming routine can address the out-of-control input circle holding us down.

5. Work on your jargon

This could appear to be unlikely, yet there is significant proof that profound granularity is firmly connected to semantic granularity. The more finely grained your jargon, the more definitively your cerebrum can distinguish what's going on in the body and align its financial plan likewise.

In a review, it was found that individuals who display higher profound granularity go to the specialist less habitually, use prescriptions less much of the time, and spend fewer days hospitalized for sickness. Interestingly, lower profound granularity is related to the significant burdensome problem, social nervousness issues, dietary issues, chemical imbalance range issues, marginal behavioral conditions, and general sensations of tension and sorrow.

Whether it is perusing modern and nuanced works of writing, watching motion pictures with complex characters, or looking into words you don't have the foggiest idea, extending your jargon can straightforwardly affect your body capability.

6. Expound on your encounters
One of the reasonable ends of How Emotions Are Made is that the universe of ideas and the universe of science are not independent. Our cerebrum depends on models of what's going on or is prone to occur in the rest of the world to settle on planning choices. We can intentionally impact and enhance these models by what we open ourselves to.

Composing is one of the best approaches to straightforwardly shape the ideas our mind is developing. Composing permits us to make our reasoning more concrete, outside our heads, where it very well may be all the more dispassionately assessed, investigated, and changed. The words we put on the page can be reflected in us, shaping an alternate prescient circle in which we have significantly more organization.

The last word

Every one of the six of these methodologies can transform a negative twisting of enduring into simple actual inconvenience. Torment is inescapable, however, it doesn't need to mean something is off about your life. No procedure is ensured to work like clockwork, however, they open up the chance of pursuing a better body, additional satisfying connections, and a more adaptable and intense close-to-home life.

The commitment of built emotions isn't that we will some way or another deal with how we feel. Emotions are innately questionable, and that vulnerability is the preciseness exact thing that makes a lively profound life conceivable. Life can be suddenly upbeat, out of the blue, significant, startlingly significant. The commitment isn't that we have some control over the profound waves that range over us as we travel through life. The commitment is that we can figure out how to ride those waves with expertise and with delight.

Chapter 3

How does your thinking affect your emotions?

Assuming somebody begins discussing what contemplations mean for emotions, the vast majority would handily grasp the idea of positive reasoning. This is with the comprehension that 'good' believing is the best way to go, and that good reasoning encourages us. Or on the other hand, in any event, better. However, are considerations and emotions as straightforward as this?

Unfortunately - this is nevertheless essential for the story! There is another side to it. In this article, I plan to address a few fundamental ideas and connections.

What are your Thoughts?
We'd all probably concur that we comprehend that contemplations are the voice inside our heads. The voice converses

with us continually. The voice expresses kind things, and it expresses frightful things. It tends to be useful and it very well may be exceptionally pointless. It very well may out and out pester! It never appears to quiet down! This is our reasoning cerebrum. Our cognizant psyche.

It is detailed that we have around 50,000 to 70,000 considerations each day. The National Science Foundation says a typical individual has around 12,000 to 60,000 considerations each day. Whichever figure is nearest to the fact of the matter, that is still a ton of contemplations!

The quantity of considerations is a certain something, yet the second piece of the story is the truly intriguing thing. All quite well assuming they are useful, positive, and elevating considerations. What's more, in so being, help by extending us towards our objectives and dreams! However, No! 80% of them are negative considerations

What Thoughts Mean for Emotions isn't New News

We needn't bother with being straight understudies to perceive that rehashing, a large number of days after day, a huge number of negative considerations, won't be something to be thankful for.

Numerous savvy men have mentioned that equivalent objective fact.

Lao Tzu was a Chinese scholar who lived from 601BC. This statement is licensed to him:

"Watch your contemplations; they become words. Watch your words; they become activities. Watch your activities; they become propensity. Watch your propensities; they become character. Watch your personality; it turns into your fate."

One of the world's most extraordinary and motivational figures, Mahatma Gandhi, who lived somewhere in the range of 1869 and 1948, has been recorded as having said:

"A man is nevertheless the result of his viewpoints. His thought process, he becomes."

(I'm certain he implied something very similar for ladies)

Eckhart Tolle, a current profound instructor, and creator (conceived 1948) said:

"The essential driver of misery is never the circumstance, however, the considerations about it, Be mindful of the contemplations you are thinking"

Thus, monitoring our considerations is extraordinarily significant assuming we wish to feel cheerful and find actual success.

Is Positive Thinking the Answer?
I'm not prescribing to just think decidedly and forever be blissful and thus live joyfully ever later! That is ludicrous! What's more, a seriously undesirable assumption to put on ourselves (as well as other people).

I am, nonetheless, committed to assisting individuals with understanding the strong impact our contemplations have on our prosperity.

To know how considerations are shaped, how we can 'manage' our contemplations, and what our contemplations mean for our emotions is to have an extraordinary understanding of our outlook.

Contemplations and Emotions
Contemplations and emotions are very unmistakable, and they are likewise inseparably related.

What are emotions?

An unmistakable inclination getting from one's conditions, state of mind, or associations with others

one more definition is given:

natural or instinctive inclination as recognized from thinking or information.

What's more, Wikipedia says:

The feeling is a psychological state related to the sensory system welcomed on by compound changes differently connected with considerations, sentiments, conduct reactions, and a level of joy or dismay. There is at present no logical agreement on a definition.

Where Does This Knowledge Come From?

It's not difficult to find out about our actual well-being, and how to oversee it. Also, it's not difficult to go off and learn ideas and information to place in our minds. Be that as it may, finding out about emotions and how to deal with them is less plainly characterized and perceived.

Since emotions can be said to control our lives, this leaves a fairly enormous hole in our life training. Unfortunate comprehension of why we respond as we do influences our capacity to oversee how we feel from one day to another!

Our emotions drive us, however, they are the things we know the most un-about.

Emotions can be welcomed by an outside episode like having a contention with a friend or family member or watching a parody show and snickering generously. Emotions can likewise be blended by something inside us, similar to a memory of a miserable or startling experience.

Everybody the world over encounters emotions. However, every individual will respond to them another way. Contingent on culture and childhood, individuals may not understand what they are feeling, or why. For instance, a few societies will communicate delight illustratively, similar to the Italians. English nobility will have been prepped to be significantly more held and controlled in the declaration of emotions.

A Helpful Way to Think of Emotions
With regards to a solid mentality, conveyed by considerations and emotions that help a supportive and fruitful point of view, an accommodating method for considering emotions is:
Energy in Motion
If we are to feel the energy of feeling and permit it to travel through the regular cycle it was expected to, then we have felt and handled the inclination.

Handling feelings in a solid manner
We watch a satire show and giggle at each joke for a couple of moments. And afterward, that joke is finished. The entertainer thinks of the following joke, we chuckle once more, and the show happens as such. We don't snicker for a long time over only one joke!

We go across the street without having seen an oncoming vehicle - and move all-powerful dismay and hop in time. Huge apprehension overwhelmed us, saved us, and filled its need. When we understand we are protected and have promised to take more consideration in the future, we recuperate from the fear. We have "handled" the inclination.

Not handling emotions
What occurs, however, in the situation where our emotions are suppressed? As a youngster

maybe we were shown it isn't more right than wrong to communicate outrage or trouble. Or on the other hand, youngsters ought to be seen and not heard, thus shouldn't talk about our considerations and thoughts in the grown-up organization. Thus, we needed to bottle outrage and misery inside. We figured out how to remain quiet about our viewpoints, similar to they are not deserving of sharing.

Suppressed emotions don't disappear. They work, with each rehashed episode. In the end, at some point, some surprising occasion will set off the arrival of a suppressed feeling. Consider suppressed outrage, bringing about savage explosions.

These packaged emotions are extremely unfortunate. There is proof to show that suppressed emotions can cause tension, discouragement, and different illnesses and medical problems.

What's more, the considerations we have, every day, can contribute - in a supportive OR pointless manner.

How Thoughts Affect Emotions
Our thought process influences what we feel. Contemplations trigger emotions. Good considerations can set off positive sentiment emotions and pessimistic contemplations can set off emotions that outcome in us feeling awful.

This shouldn't imply that all emotions that cause us to feel terrible are off-base, or awful in themselves. For instance, if we have lost a friend or family member, we want to feel miserable. That is correct and normal.

Yet, feeling furious, miserable, or unfortunate (or an entire host of different emotions) because of considerations that are not practical to the circumstance isn't the best thing to manage. Especially as long as possible.

Channel what enters our faculties
A model is watching the information. What stories are forthcoming in the information? The awful ones. The miserable ones. The startling ones. They catch individuals' eyes and that is the thing the news source means to do. They need watchers and they need to introduce the news in a manner that stands out for quite a while.

Another model is investing energy in overly critical, angry, individual discussions in a disparaging, irate, or offending way. What considerations will focus on this?

Assuming we permit our psyches to be loaded up with unfortunate, monstrous, furious, and troubling messages, almost certainly, our considerations will be impacted by that to some extent. While perhaps not right away, then an eating routine of such a mental siege can cause significant damage over the long run.

A shortfall of supportive, steady, and positive effects on our viewpoints vows to convey a truly hopeless point of view.

With the ascent of sadness and tension, upsetting degrees of abusive behavior at home, and self-destruction in our general public, it appears to be like any consideration given to dealing with our viewpoints is a positive methodology.

(Note: not the slightest bit am I proposing placing our heads in the sand and disregarding reality! I'm proposing a standpoint of equilibrium and point of view.)

Could we at any point Choose our Thoughts and Emotions?
Indeed, by and large, we can.

With a wish to all the more likely deal with our outlook and emotional wellness, in addition to the right tool stash and direction, we can.

Furthermore, this is the reason and expectation behind my reality as an outlook guide. Having taken myself from somebody who had no information on the impact of contemplations on emotions, and was fairly a heap of tension, I completely value the phenomenal power this groundbreaking data can have on an individual's life! Assuming you wish to find how to make your universe of quiet, expanded clearness, decreased pressure, and better progress in all parts of your life.

Chapter 4

Solutions to negative emotions

The capacity to experience and communicate emotions is a higher priority than you could understand.

As the felt reaction to a given circumstance, emotions have a critical impact on your responses. At the point when you're on top of them, you approach significant information that assists with:

navigation

relationship achievement

everyday corporations

taking care of oneself

While emotions can play a supportive part in your routine, they can negatively affect your close-to-home well-being and relational connections when they begin to feel wild.

Vicki Botnick, a specialist in Tarzana, California, makes sense that any inclination, even delight, bliss, or others you'd commonly consider positive — can escalate to where it becomes hard to control.

With just enough practice, however, you can reclaim the rules. Two examinations from 2010Trusted Source propose that having great profound guideline abilities are connected to prosperity. Furthermore, the subsequent one tracked down a likely connection between these abilities and monetary achievement, so investing some energy on that front may in a real sense pay off.

Here are a few pointers to kick you off.

1. Investigate the effect of your emotions
Extraordinary emotions aren't all terrible.

"Emotions make our lives energizing, one of a kind, and dynamic," Botnick says. "Overwhelming inclinations can mean that we embrace life completely, that we're not stifling our normal responses."

It's completely common to encounter some profound overpowering now and again — when something superb occurs, when something horrible occurs, when you feel like you've passed up a major opportunity.

All in all, how do you have any idea when there's an issue?

Emotions that consistently go crazy could prompt:

relationship or companionship struggle
trouble connecting with others
an inconvenience at work or school
a desire to utilize substances to assist with dealing with your emotions
physical or close-to-home eruptions

Set aside an opportunity to check out exactly what your uncontrolled emotions are meaning to your everyday life. This will make it more straightforward to distinguish trouble spots (and track your prosperity).

2. Go for the gold, constraint
You have no control over your emotions with a dial (if by some stroke of good luck it were simply simple!). However, envision, briefly, that you could deal with emotions along these lines.

You would have zero desire to leave them running at greatest constantly. You likewise would have no desire to turn them off altogether, all things considered.

At the point when you stifle or curb emotions, you're keeping yourself from encountering and communicating sentiments.

This can happen deliberately (concealment) or unwittingly (restraint).

Either can add to mental and actual well-being side effects, including:

uneasiness
despondency
rest issues
muscle pressure and torment
trouble overseeing pressure
substance abuse
While figuring out how to practice command over emotions, ensure you're not simply hiding them away from plain view. Solid close-to-home articulation includes discovering a few harmonies between overpowering emotions and no emotions by any stretch of the imagination.

3. Distinguish what you're feeling

Pausing for a minute to check in with yourself about your state of mind can assist you with starting to restore control.

Let's assume you've been seeing somebody for a couple of months. You had a go at arranging a date last week, however, they said they lacked opportunity and willpower. Once more, recently, you messaged, saying, "I might want to see you soon. Might you at any point meet this week?"

They at long last answer, over a day after the fact: "Can't. Occupied."

You're unexpectedly very disturbed. Ceaselessly to think, you fling your telephone across the room, push over your wastebasket, and kick your work area, slamming your toe.

Interfere with yourself by inquiring:

What am I feeling at present? (frustrated, befuddled, angry)

What ended up causing me to feel such? (They forgot about me for no obvious reason.)

Does what is happening have an alternate clarification that could seem OK? (Perhaps they're anxious, wiped out, or managing something different they feel awkward making sense of. They could want to make more sense of more when they can.)

What is it that I believe should do about these sentiments? (Shout, vent my dissatisfaction by tossing things, text back something impolite.)

Is there a superior approach to adapting to them? (Inquire as to whether all is Well. Ask when they're free straightaway. Take a walk or run.)

By taking into account potential other options, you're rethinking your considerations, which can assist you with altering your most memorable outrageous response.

It can require some investment before this reaction turns into a propensity. With work, going through these means in your mind will become simpler (and more powerful).

4. Acknowledge your emotions — every one of them
Assuming that you're attempting to get better at dealing with emotions, you could have a go at making light of your sentiments to yourself.

At the point when you hyperventilate after getting uplifting news or breakdown on the floor shouting and wailing when you can't find your keys, it could appear to be useful to tell yourself, "Simply quiet down," or "It isn't so huge of an arrangement, so don't blow a gasket."

Yet, this negates your experience. It is nothing to joke about for you.

By tolerating emotions you become more familiar with them. Expanding your solace around extraordinary emotions permits you to completely feel them without responding in outrageous, pointless ways.

To work on tolerating emotions, have a go at considering them, couriers. They're "bad" or "awful." They're unbiased. Perhaps they raise terrible sentiments some of the time, yet they're giving you significant data that you can utilize.

For instance, attempt:

"I'm vexed because I continue to lose my keys, which makes me late. I ought to put a

dish on the rack by the entryway so I make sure to leave them in a similar spot."
Tolerating emotions might lead to trusted Sources more noteworthy life fulfillment and fewer psychological wellness side effects. Also, individuals considering their emotions accommodating may lead to trusted Sources with more significant levels of satisfaction.

5. Keep a mindset diary
Recording on paper (or composing up) your sentiments and the reactions they trigger can assist you with revealing any troublesome examples.

In some cases, sufficiently it's to follow emotions back through your viewpoints intellectually. Putting sentiments onto paper can permit you to profoundly consider them more.

It additionally assists you with perceiving when explicit conditions, similar to inconvenience at work or family struggle, add to more diligently to get a grip on emotions. Recognizing explicit triggers makes it conceivable to think of ways of overseeing them all the more gainfully.

Journaling gives the most advantage when you do it day to day. Keep your diary with you and scribble down extreme emotions or sentiments as they occur. Attempt to take note of the triggers and your response. If your response didn't help, utilize your diary to investigate more accommodating opportunities for what's to come.

6. Take a full breath
There's a lot to be said for the force of a full breath, whether you're incredibly cheerful or so irate you can't talk.

Dialing back and focusing on your breath won't make the emotions disappear (and recall, that is not the objective).

In any case, profound breathing activities can assist you with establishing yourself and making a stride back from the principal extraordinary blaze of feeling and any outrageous response you need to keep away from.

The following time you feel emotions beginning to assume command:

Take it leisurely. Full breaths come from the stomach, not the chest. It might assist with picturing your breath ascending from somewhere down in your midsection.
Hold it. Pause your breathing for a count of three, then let it out leisurely.

Think about a mantra. Certain individuals find it supportive to rehash a mantra, similar to "I'm quiet" or "I'm loose."

7. Know when to articulate your thoughts

There's an appropriate setting for everything, including extreme emotions. Wailing wildly is a typical reaction to losing a friend or family member, for instance. Shouting into your cushion, in any event, punching it, could assist you with alleviating a few outrage and strain in the wake of being unloaded.

Different circumstances, in any case, require some limitations. Regardless of how disappointed you are, shouting at your supervisor over an unreasonable disciplinary activity won't help.

Being aware of your environmental factors and the circumstance can help you realize when it's OK to let sentiments and when you should sit with them for the occasion.

8. Give yourself some space

Getting some separation from extraordinary sentiments can assist you with ensuring you're responding to them in sensible ways, as per Botnick.

This distance may be physical, such as leaving what is happening, for instance. Be that as it may, you can likewise make some psychological distance by diverting yourself.

While you would rather not block or stay away from sentiments completely, it's not destructive to divert yourself until you're in a superior spot to manage them. Simply get back into the game with them. Solid interruptions are short-lived.

Attempt:

going for a stroll

watching an entertaining video

conversing with a friend or family member

putting in no time flat with your pet

9. Attempt contemplation

Assuming you practice contemplation as of now, it very well may be one of your go-to strategies for adapting to outrageous sentiments.

Reflection can assist you with expanding your consciousness of all sentiments and encounters. At the point when you think, you're helping yourself to sit with those sentiments, to see them without passing judgment on yourself or endeavoring to change them or make them disappear.

As referenced above, figuring out how to acknowledge each of your emotions can make profound guidelines more straightforward. Contemplation assists you with expanding those acknowledgment abilities. It additionally offers different advantages, such as aiding you to unwind and get better rest.

Our manual for various types of reflection can assist you with getting everything rolling.

10. Keep steady under overpressure

At the point when you're under a great deal of pressure, dealing with your emotions can turn out to be more troublesome. Indeed, even individuals who for the most part have some control over their emotions well could track down it harder amid high strain and stress. Lessening pressure, or tracking down additional accommodating ways of overseeing it, can assist your emotions with turning out to be more sensible.

Care rehearses like contemplation can assist with pressure, as well. They will not dispose of it, yet they can make it more straightforward to live with.

Other sound ways of adapting to pressure include:

getting sufficient rest
making time to talk (and giggle) with companions
work out
spending

11. Converse with a specialist
If your emotions keep on feeling overpowering, it could be an ideal opportunity to look for proficient help.
Long haul or diligent profound dysregulation and emotional episodes are connected to specific psychological wellness conditions, including marginal behavioral conditions and bipolar issues. Inconvenience controlling emotions can likewise connect with injury,

family issues, or other fundamental worries, which Botnick makes sense of.

A specialist can offer merciful, without judgment support as you:

investigate factors adding to dysregulated emotions

address serious emotional episodes

figure out how down-control serious sentiments or up-direct restricted profound articulation

work on testing and reexamining sentiments that cause trouble

Temperament swings and extreme emotions can incite pessimistic or undesirable considerations that ultimately trigger sensations of sadness or depression.

This cycle can ultimately prompt pointless survival strategies like self-mischief or even considerations of self-destruction. If you start pondering self-destruction or have desires to self-hurt, converse with a believed cherished one who can assist you with moving help immediately.